Essential Oils Book

40 Recipes for Children

Table of Contents

Introduction

I would first like to thank and congratulate you on downloading *"Essential Oils for Kids"* As parents we naturally want the best for our children, with that in mind I decided to put together this book of essential oil recipes that are safe for kids. Many people today are seeking the natural products over synthetic chemical filled products. We as parents feel much better in knowing the products that we are using with our children are not filled with harmful chemicals. We feel good in knowing the natural products are instead offering them health benefits that are natural and safe.

Not only can you secure in using natural products such as essential oils with your children, but using "green" environmentally friendly natural products gives you a sense that you are doing your part in keeping our planet green. Using environmentally friendly products with your children is teaching your children a very vital and important lesson in how to live without harming the environment that they live in—their home. Important lessons indeed for your children to learn, eventually they will pass these important lessons learned onto the next generation and so forth. One of the best ways to teach our children a healthy way to live is certainly by example. Children look up to their parents (adults in their lives) for guidance, it is up to us to do our part to make sure that we are putting forth the right kind of message through the examples we set. Teaching our kids how to use essential oils that offer multipurpose uses is a great start to teaching them some environmentally friendly choices in their lives.

Chapter 1. What Are Essential Oils?

Using a form of distillation the natural essential oils are collected from various plants, quite often they contain the fragrance of the plant from which the oils were collected. Essential oils have been part of human history for thousands of years. They have been used in many natural health treatments, beauty treatments, aromatherapy and household cleaners.

More people are choosing to use homemade products or natural products that include essential oil rather than using products that are not environmentally safe and are filled with harsh chemicals.

People like that essential oil products do not have the severe side effects of synthetic products. People are becoming more aware and concerned about the kinds of unnatural additives that are being added into their products that they use on themselves and in their homes. Knowing that natural products are the more healthier choice more people are choosing them over synthetic products. People are also becoming more aware of things that we can do that are environmentally friendly such as using natural products instead of synthetic ones. As parents we certainly want to choose products that are safe to use on and around our children.

Safety Tips when Using Essential Oils

1. Use a base oil such as olive oil when using essential oils. Base oils are known as "carrier oils" they are used with essential oils due to essential oils be very concentrated. It is best to dilute essential oils before using them.

2. Store essential oils in a cool location away from light. If you store essential oils properly they will maintain their potency for many years.

3. Make sure to keep them out of reach of small children. With children under the age of 30 months do not use peppermint essential oil around their throat area.

4. Keep essential oils away from eyes and ears.

5. Pregnant women should consult with their health care provider before using essential oils. They should not use constituents that have hormone-like activity such as juniper, sage, clary sage, fennel and Idaho tansy.

6. People that suffer from epilepsy should avoid using essential oils especially fennel, hyssop, and Idaho tansy. It is best for them to consult their health care provider.

7. If you are someone that suffers from allergies it is a good idea to do a small test patch on your skin to see how you react to essential oils. A safe area to apply essential oils is on the feet.

8. Before ingesting essential oils make sure that they are "GRAS" (generally regarded as safe) and dilute them with a base oil such as olive oil.

9. Do not add essential oils that have not been diluted to your bath water. They will not dilute directly in bath water, first dilute them with a base oil of your choice.

10. You will find that many of my essential oil recipes request the use of spray bottles or containers for storing essential oils products. The best containers to store them in are glass dark containers.

The above tips or suggested uses only apply to Therapeutic grade, young living essential oils.

General Supplies

- **Carrier oils**—use these oils to dilute your essential oils.

- **Castile soap**—this is basic simple soap with no chelating agents, dyes, whiteners, or synthetic fragrances.

- **Citric Acid**—is a natural occurring acid in fruits, it helps increase bacterial environment, making it very difficult for microbes to survive, it is a great addition to home cleaning products.

- **Distilled White Vinegar**—it is great to use as a cleaning product due to its high acidity content. Great to use in neutralizing odors.

- **Glycerin**—it is used to thicken many skin care and moisturizer recipes.

- **Shea butter**—it has fatty acids and a concentration of natural vitamins that help nourish skin. It also has anti-inflammatory properties offering healing benefits.

- **Washing Soda**—it is a great product for washing that is not filled with unnatural chemicals and is inexpensive to use.

- **Beeswax**—it offers a number of benefits, including anti-inflammatory properties that can help calm and soothe.

- **Baking soda**—it can help eliminate odors and is a "green" cleaning agent.

Chapter 2. Kid Friendly Essential Oils Recipe Collection

1. *Glowing Skin with Patchouli*

Ingredients:

- shampoo or lotion
- 4 drops Patchouli essential oil

Directions:

Add in the Patchouli essential oil in with your child's shampoo or skin lotion and blend well. You will soon notice the hue of their skin will improve with regular use.

2. *Lemongrass Fungus Killer*

Ingredients:

- 4 drops Lemongrass essential oil
- 1 teaspoon of distilled water

Directions:

Add the lemongrass essential oil drops to 1 teaspoon of water and stir. Apply this solution to your child's skin using a cotton swab. Your child's skin will be fungus-free in no time.

3. *Build Confidence with Tangerine*

Ingredients:

- 1 drop of tangerine essential oil

- 8 ounces of water or juice

Directions:

Add one drop of tangerine essential oil to your child's juice or water in the morning. You may also choose to add 2 drops to their water at night. Tangerine essential oil will help keep your child calm. It works well with children that are nervous or shy. Taking a dose of it before bed will allow them to sleep and wake up feeling totally energized and refreshed.

4. *Frankincense to Keep Skin Healthy*

Ingredients:

- 1 drop Frankincense essential oil

- 16 ounces of water

Directions:

Add the Frankincense to 16 ounces of water and have your child drink this once a day. It offers many healing properties it can ingested or used topically. Add a few drops in shampoo and skin lotions as well to keep child's skin and hair healthy. Add to a diffuser to offer a nice rich scent to the room, it pairs well with other essential oils such as sandalwood, cedar or tea tree.

5. Relax Child Using Sandalwood

Ingredients:

- 2 drops sandalwood essential oil

- 8 ounces of water

- 1 tablespoon organic honey

Directions:

In an 8 ounce glass of warm water add in sandalwood essential oil and honey then stir. Give to child to drink, this will help them to relax. They will be able to sleep, and this will also soothe sore throat.

6. Citrus Energizer

Ingredients:

- 2 drops citrus essential oil

- 8 ounces water or juice

Directions:

Add to your child's juice or water the citrus essential oil in the morning. This will help your child to feel energized to start their day. It will help child stay focused and energized.

7. *Fighting Allergies with Rose Otto*

Ingredients:

- 3 drops Rose Otto essential oil

- 8 ounce glass juice or water

Directions:

In the morning add a couple of drops of Rose Otto essential oil to your child's juice. Add a few drops into a diffuser in your home. You will notice in no time that your child will gain relief from bothersome allergies. Using this will not cause your child to feel weighed down with drowsiness. Rose Otto is not allergen specific, it can be used for air borne allergies, whether they are pollen or pet dander or others. Add a few drops to diffuser, and your child will stop sniffling in no time.

8. *St John's Wart as a Pain Killer*

Ingredients:

- 3 drops St John's Wart essential oil

- 8 ounce glass water or juice

Directions:

Add St John's Wart to the juice or glass of water and give to your child. You can also burn a few drops in an oil warmer in your child's bedroom at night just before bedtime. The aroma will have an effect like a sedative and will cause your child to drift off into a peaceful sleep. It is also known for helping to treat ear aches.

9. *Grapefruit Essential Oil Antiseptic & Antioxidant*

Ingredients:

- 2 drops Grapefruit essential oil

- 8 ounces of lemonade or juice

Directions:

Add essential oil to child's juice. This remedy is great to use during cold and flu season, it will boost your child's immune system. It is also great to use as an antiseptic on wounds or abrasions on your child. It will kill germs and sooth, it will not irritate the injury.

10. *Using Saffron for Aches & Pains*

Ingredients:

- 4 drops Saffron essential oil

- 1 tablespoon almond oil

Directions:

Blend these oils and then apply to the area of body where aches and pains are. It works as a good remedy for fever as well, just spread it across your child's forehead.

11. *Nail Soak for Children*

Ingredients:

- 3 drops lemon essential oil

- small dish warm water

Directions:

Fill a small dish with warm water and add in lemon essential oil and mix. Have your child soak their nails in the bowl of solution. This will treat thin and peeling nails.

12. *Helping Child to Focus with Rosemary*

Ingredients:

- 1 drop of Rosemary essential oil

- 1 teaspoon of water

Directions:

You can use rosemary essential oil to help your child to stay focused. Before your child leaves for school dip your finger in this solution and spread it across your child's forehead. It will help to keep your child focused and driven through their morning. You can use this yourself to help you to remain focused on work.

13. Cold/Sinus Infection Fighter with Eucalyptus

Ingredients:

- 4 drops of Eucalyptus essential oil

- 8 ounce glass orange juice

Directions:

Add the Eucalyptus essential oil drops into glass of orange juice and stir. Give this to your child to drink, this will help heal a sinus infection or cold.

14. Tummy Pain Relief using Red Mandarin

Ingredients:

- 4 drops of Red Mandarin essential oil

- small amount of warm water

Directions:

In a bowl of warm water add in the Red Mandarin essential oil and blend. Use a facecloth to soak up the mix and apply to your child's abdomen. Your child should soon feel relief of any abdomen pain they are feeling. It can be used for headaches or body aches.

15. Anti-diarrhoea Recipe using Cinnamon

Ingredients:

- 20 drops of cinnamon essential oil

- 8 ounces of water, tea, milk—any beverage your child likes to drink

Directions:

In an eight ounce glass beverage add in the 20 drops of cinnamon essential oil, do this three times a day. Using this recipe will stave off salmonella and other food borne illness.

16. Tummy Ache Reliever using Peppermint

Ingredients:

- 4 drops of peppermint essential oil

- 8 ounces preferred drink of your child's

Directions:

Add the 4 drops of peppermint into child's drink just before bedtime, this remedy will help to keep digestion flowing regularly and will ease tummy pain.

17. *Room Deodorizer that is Kid Friendly*

Ingredients:

- 1 teaspoon of witch hazel

- 20 drops of Purification essential oil

- 4 ounces of distilled water

Directions:

Add the above ingredients into a spray bottle. Shake before each use, spraying on fabric and in rooms.

18. *Kid Friendly Carpet Deodorizer*

Ingredients:

- 2 cups of baking soda

- 10 drops lemon essential oil

- 10 drops Purification essential oil

Directions:

Mix essential oils and baking soda until they are free of clumps. Place in old cheese shaker. Shake the mix over your carpets and leave on for 20 minutes. Vacuum up after 20 minutes, it will get rid of odors in carpet.

19. Fun Fizzy Bathroom Bomb

Ingredients:

- 1 teaspoon carrier oil such as almond oil

- 8 ounces of baking soda

- 4 ounces of corn starch

- few drops of food coloring

- 30 drops of essential oil lavender or other preferred essential oil to use in bath

- 3/4 teaspoons of water

- 4 ounces of citric acid

Directions:

Add all of your dry ingredients into a bowl and whisk. In another bowl combine wet ingredients. Add wet ingredients to dry ingredients and mix. Pack tightly into molds. Leave in molds for a few minutes then remove from molds and store in container that is airtight.

20. Bath Bombs

Ingredients:

- 4 ounces corn starch

- 6 ounces citric acid

- 4 ounces Epsom salts

- a few drops of food coloring

- 1 teaspoon of carrier oil such as almond oil

- 10 drops each of peppermint, lemon, lavender essential oils

- 8 ounces of baking soda

Directions:

Mix dry ingredients in bowl. Mix wet ingredients in bowl. Add wet ingredients to dry and mix well. Add to molds and pack well. Leave in molds for a few minutes then carefully remove bath bombs and place in airtight container.

21. Nodding-Off Bedtime Rub

Ingredients:

- 12 drops of Frankincense essential oil

- 12 drops of Vetiver essential oil

- 10 drops of lavender essential oil

- 1/4 cup of cocoa butter

- 1/4 cup of coconut oil

Directions:

Heat cocoa butter in a small pan, and coconut oil over low heat until they are melted. Removing pan from heat allow to cool, add in essential oils and mix. Place in fridge for an hour. Remove from fridge and mix solution with hand mixer until it forms peaks. Apply this to your child's feet.

22. Kid Friendly Stain Remover

Ingredients:

- 3 tablespoons of Castile soap

- 20 drops of essential oil

- 1/3 cup of hydrogen peroxide (3%)

Directions:

Mix your ingredients in a bowl, add them into a dark glass spray bottle. Both the lemon and hydrogen peroxide are sensitive to light so store in a dark place to keep potency of stain remover. Spray on stain and allow it to sit there for 5 minutes then rinse while rubbing fabric.

23. *Detangler for Kids Tangles*

Ingredients:

- 5 drops of lavender essential oil
- 5 drops of peppermint essential oil
- 2 cups of distilled water
- 1/2 cup of YL conditioner

Directions:

Bring water to a simmer. Add water and conditioner mix into a spray bottle. Add in the essential oils and shake. Apply detangler to child's hair as needed. You can leave it in or rinse it out.

24. *Gentle Laundry Detergent*

Ingredients:

- 3 cups of borax
- 30 drops of essential oil such as lemon, lavender and Purification
- 2 bars of Castile soap
- 3 cups baking soda
- 3 cups washing soda

Directions:

Mix in bowl borax, baking soda, washing soda. Use a cheese grater for soap, place into food processor along with powdered mix. Allow the mixer to blend contents. Add in essential oils and add mix to a 1 gallon container. This recipe will make 1 gallon of detergent that will be good for 125 loads.

Tip: Add 1-2 teaspoons of white vinegar as a natural fabric softener.

25. *Apple Teething Biscuit*

Ingredients:

- 1 teaspoon of baking powder

- 1 cup of rolled oats

- 1 cup of steel oats

- 1 cup of organic apple sauce, unsweetened

- 2 tablespoons of maple syrup

- 2 tablespoons of coconut oil

- 1/2 teaspoon ginger, vanilla extract, nutmeg, and cinnamon

- 10 drops each of copaiba and lavender essential oils

Directions:

Mix dry ingredients, add in syrup, essential oils, and melted coconut oil. Form shapes that are date-like and place onto a greased baking sheet. Bake at 350° Fahrenheit for 45 minutes, halfway through flip biscuits.

26. *Calming Balm for Kids*

Ingredients:

- 10 drops Frankincense essential oil

- 20 drops lavender essential oil

- 2 ounces of your choice of carrier oil such as almond oil

- 3/4 ounce beeswax

- 1 ounce Shea butter

Directions:

Melt the Shea butter and beeswax, in pan over medium heat and stir until it has melted. Remove mix from heat and pour into tin container, add in essential oils and mix. This is great for using after a bath or just before bedtime to help promote a nice calm and restful sleep for your child.

27. Bottom Soother

Ingredients:

- 3/4 cup of Shea butter
- 3 drops of Frankincense essential oil
- 4 drops lavender essential oil
- 1/4 cup coconut oil

Directions:

In a bowl whip your Shea butter and coconut oil with hand mixer. Add in the essential oils and whip once more. Keep mixing until the mix has a nice frosting-like texture to it. This can be great at helping soothe diaper rash, and other skin irritations.

28. DIY Simple Bubble Bath

Ingredients:

- 1 cup of liquid Castile soap
- 1/2 cup of Glycerin
- 13 drops of lavender essential oil
- 4 tablespoons of water

Directions:

Mix ingredients in a glass bottle and shake well before each use.

29. *Chest Rub for Kids*

Ingredients:

- 3 tablespoons of coconut oil

- 1 tablespoon of beeswax

- 30 drops of RC essential oil

Directions:

Place a small glass jar into a pot of water. Add in beeswax, coconut oil in jar. Heat up pot until beeswax and coconut oil have melted. Remove from heat add in the essential oils and mix well. Keep in fridge.

30. *Oil for Outchies*

Ingredients:

- 10 drops of lavender essential oil

- 10 drops of Frankincense essential oil

- witch hazel

- carrier oil such as olive oil

Directions:

Add ingredients into a roller bottle, made of glass. Shake well before each use. Apply solution to cuts, rashes, scrapes and bites.

31. *Slimy Slime*

Ingredients:

- 1 cup of liquid starch

- food coloring

- 4 tablespoons of glitter

- 2 bottles of clear school glue

- 5 drops of essential oil of choice from this selection: lavender, lemon,

Directions:

Add bottles of glue to a bowl, add in essential oil and mix. Add in the food coloring and liquid starch and mix. Leave it to sit in a ball for a few minutes. Knead ball until it is nice and slimy.

32. *Tuner for Tummy*

Ingredients:

- carrier oil such as olive oil or almond oil

- 6-8 drops of DiGize essential oil

Directions:

Apply this mix directly on to tummy or on bottom of feet. You can use this on children, pets and adults. Add mix in a roller bottle. Shake before each use.

33. *Sparkling Play Dough made with Essential Oil*

Ingredients:

- 20 drops of essential oil choose from: StressAway, Thieves, lemon, lavender
- 2 cups of almond flour
- 4 tablespoons of silver glitter
- 3/4 cup of carrier oil of your choice
- 1 cup of corn starch
- food coloring

Directions:

Mix all ingredients in bowl. Knead the mix and store in an airtight container.

34. *Regular Play Dough made with Essential Oil*

Ingredients:

- 2 cups of almond flour
- 20 drops of essential oil choose from: lavender, lemon, StessAway, and Thieves
- 2 tablespoons of carrier oil
- 2 tablespoons of cream of tartar
- food coloring
- 1 1/2 cups boiling water
- 1/2 cup table salt

Directions:

In a bowl add cream of tartar, flour, salt, carrier oil. Add in the boiling water and mix it until dough forms. Add in the food coloring and mix. Knead the dough adding in the essential oil. Store in airtight container.

35. *Kid Friendly Bug Spray*

Ingredients:

- 50 drops of essential oils choose from: citronella, lemongrass, mint, lavender, tea tree, rosemary, purification and Thieves

- top off with witch hazel

- 1/2 bottle of distilled water

Directions:

Add all of the ingredients in a spray bottle and shake well before each use.

36. *Oil for Scars*

Ingredients:

- 10 drops of lavender essential oil

- carrier oil of your choice

- 5 drops of Purification essential oil

- 5 drops of Frankincense essential oil

Directions:

Add all of the ingredients into a spray bottle and apply to scared areas of your child's skin such as bug bites, rashes and scrapes.

37. *Hair & Body Wash for Kids*

Ingredients:

- 10 drops of StressAway essential oil
- 10 drops of orange essential oil
- 1 cup of Castile soap
- distilled water
- 1 teaspoon of aloe vera juice
- 1 tablespoon of carrier oil
- 2 tablespoons of glycerin

Directions:

Add Castile soap, essential oils, glycerin, aloe vera juice to a pump bottle. Top this mix off with distilled water. Add and secure the lid, shake well before each use.

38. *Body Scrub for Kids*

Ingredients:

- 1 cup of coconut oil
- 1/2 cup of Castile soap
- 2 cups of corse sugar or salt
- 5 drops of peppermint essential oil

- 5 drops of lavender essential oil

- 5 drops of Frankincense essential oil

Directions:

Add the carrier oil such as suggested coconut oil in recipe into bowl. Add in sugar or salt and mix. This will make a great scrub for hands and feet of your child, keep in mason jar.

39. Citrus Strawberry Popsicles

Ingredients:

- 2 pints of strawberries, fresh, hulled, sliced

- 4 drops of lemon essential oil

- 2 drops of lime essential oil

- 1/2 cup of water

- 1/2 cup of evaporated cane juice crystals

- 1/8 teaspoon of sea salt, fine

Directions:

In a pan add in your cane juice crystals, strawberries, water and bring these to a boil over medium heat, then reduce to a simmer. Once your crystals have completely dissolved remove from the heat. Add in the lime and lemon essential oils after mix is cooked and removed from heat. Add ingredients into your food processor and blend mix until nice and smooth. Add this into your Popsicle molds and leave them in freezer overnight. The next day your child can enjoy this healthy treat!

40. Orange Popsicles

Ingredients:

- 1 cup of water

- 2 cups of NingXia Red

- 7 drops of orange essential oil

Directions:

Mix all of your ingredients in a bowl then add them into Popsicle molds and leave in freezer overnight and the next day your child will have a great healthy treat to enjoy!

Conclusion

I hope that you and your loved ones will enjoy making and using my collection of essential oil based recipes for kids. You can have a lot of fun with your child making these recipes up and teaching them at the same time how to make healthier choices. Take the time to explain to them how making their own homemade products is much better not just for them but for the environment! Teach to your child how important it is to take care of themselves and their surroundings, and of course one of the best ways to do this is by example. Showing your child is going to teach them some wonderful and valuable lessons that they will be able to take with them when it comes time for them to leave the nest. They in turn will someday teach their own children how to prepare natural essential oil based home solutions and remedies.

You can feel good in knowing that you have taught and provided your child with solutions and remedies that will offer them great benefits in life. Our children need to be given the best and healthiest treatments that we can offer them. Offering them homemade natural products is definitely a good choice. We can feel good in knowing that they will not be filled with all kinds of artificial additives, and chemicals. As parents we try and give the best to our children that we can offer them, knowing we are giving them natural products is definitely a good healthy choice that we can make for our children.

I wish to thank you once again for downloading my book and supporting my work. It is very important to me that I am giving my readers what they want. I would love to read a review by you of my book in Amazon. Have fun making and using my kids collection of essential oil based recipes!

FREE Bonus Reminder

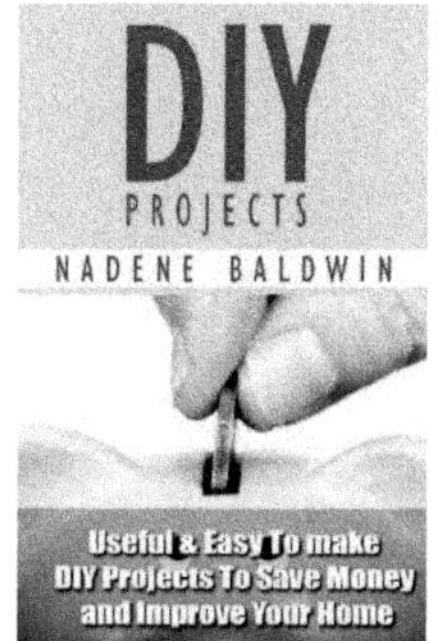

If you have not grabbed it yet, please go ahead and download your special bonus report *"DIY Projects. 13 Useful & Easy To Make DIY Projects To Save Money & Improve Your Home!"*
Simply Click the Button Below

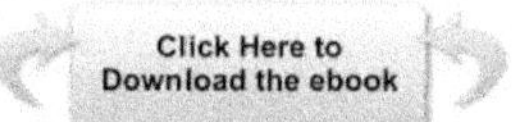

OR **Go to This Page**
http://diyhomecraft.com/free

BONUS #2: More Free & Discounted Books or Products
Do you want to receive more Free/Discounted Books or Products?
We have a mailing list where we send out our new Books or Products when they go free or with a discount on Amazon. Click on the link below to sign up for Free & Discount Book & Product Promotions.
=> Sign Up for Free & Discount Book & Product Promotions <=

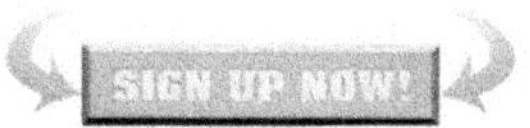

OR Go to this URL
http://zbit.ly/1WBb1Ek